COURAGEOUS NEW DAWN

HEALING VERSES – POETRY NAVIGATING PAIN,
EMOTION, AND RENEWED STRENGTH IN 50+ SHADES
OF FEELINGS

WHAT TO DO FIRST SERIES!
BOOK TWO

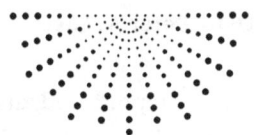

PETER A LAST

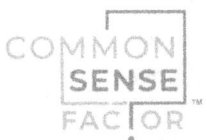

Published by CS Factor Book Publishing
Copyright © 2023 1206046 by Peter A. Last
All rights reserved.
No part of this publication may be reproduced, distributed, or transmitted in any form or by any means, including photocopying, recording, or other electronic or mechanical methods, without the prior written permission of the publisher, except in the case of brief quotations embodied in critical reviews and specific other non-commercial uses permitted by copyright law. For permission requests, write to the publisher, addressed "Attention: Permissions Coordinator," at the address below.

CS Factor Book Publishing
admin@csfactor.com
Publishing Manager/Author: P. Last
ISBN 978-1-7380495-0-9 E-Book
ISBN 978-1-7380495-1-6 Audio
ISBN 978-1-7380495-2-3 Paperback
ISBN 978-1-7380495-3-0 Hard Cover

Man Set Impressions

"Within the societal impressions set by man, especially during the Industrial Revolution, a culture emerged where suppressing emotions became a tool for increased productivity. It's time to break free from these constructed norms and embrace our true selves."

— COMMON SENSE FACTOR

This book is a dedication to the men and women of the world who have been molded by fear and anxiety, influencing who they are and how they interact with the world. It is a call to all men and women who may feel disconnected from their emotions and disconnected from their true desires. We have been programmed to follow a safe and steady path handed down to us from previous generations. We have been taught not to show emotion or vulnerability, which may reflect weakness. But at what cost? Many of us have experienced childhood traumas that affect our confidence and ability to express ourselves fully. We hold in our feelings, not realizing that our emotions are essential to our being.

We must allow ourselves to feel, to express ourselves, and to embrace our true desires. It takes strength to acknowledge our fears and vulnerabilities and courage to confront them.

It's time to break the cycle of non-emotional responses and limitations ingrained in us for generations. We must let go of the fear of being judged as weak or vulnerable and understand that it is okay to show emotion. By confronting our anxieties and traumas, we can begin to heal and live a life filled with joy, purpose, and connection.

So, to all the men and women, understand that your fear and anxiety do not define you. It's time to be direct and firm as we confront our emotions and embrace our true selves. Let us break free from the limiting belief system and strive for a life filled with happiness and fulfillment.

PREFACE

Courageous New Dawn

In a world once veiled in uncertain haze,
Where shadows of fear cast long, dark days,
Comes a beacon, a hope, a courageous new dawn,
Signaling to us all: It's time to move on.
In the still of the night, when anxieties stir,
Echoes of the past, a world that once was,
Rise above the whispers, the echoes of doubt,
Mastering your mindset is what life's about.
Fear, a foe familiar, dressed in disguise,
Tells tales of despair beneath starry skies,
Yet within every heart, there lies a flame,
It is the power to overcome, to rewrite the game.
Conquer anxiety, that thief in the night,
With wisdom and courage, with innermost light,

For even in darkness, one truth remains clear,
The power to thrive is stronger than fear.
Post-pandemic memories, some bitter, some sweet,
Have taught us resilience and made us complete.
Embrace every lesson; let not one be in vain,
For through every storm, there's wisdom to gain.
Now, stand at the brink of a world reborn,
Embrace the challenges, the thorns, and the born,
For with every sunrise, a promise is made,
Of a courageous new dawn, where hopes never fade.
Master your thoughts, let them dance, let them soar,
For in the heart of the brave, fear is no more.
Thriving and shining in a world so grand,
With the power of mindset, together we stand.

— P LAST

INTRODUCTION

Fear and Anxiety are soul messages to be listened to!

— COMMON SENSE FACTOR

In the twilight of our collective ordeal, as the world gingerly stepped out of the shadows of a global pandemic, we have come to recognize a truth: the scars that such monumental experiences leave behind are not just physical or societal but deeply emotional and psychological. The journey from fear to freedom, from anxiety to assurance, is as intricate as the winding paths of our minds.

"Courageous New Dawn" endeavors to be the candle that lights up these paths. This collection is an anthology of poems and a therapeutic companion for the heart and soul. Each poem is a meditation, a mantra, a reflection on a particular emotion that has come to the forefront in this post-pandemic world. Through verses, we will confront our fears, challenge our anxieties, and chart a course toward a brighter, more resilient future.

Every emotion, every shadow, every ray of hope finds its voice here. These are poems for the brave, those who dare to face their innermost feelings head-on, and those who are determined to emerge stronger, wiser, and more compassionate. In mastering our mindset, we find personal healing and contribute to recovering the world around us.

So, as you turn the pages, allow yourself to feel, to resonate, and to embark on the transformative journey of "Courageous New Dawn." Let these verses be the whispers of encouragement, the balm for your spirit, and the catalyst for your inner child revolution. Welcome to a poetic odyssey of resilience, recovery, and rebirth.

If you get inspired while reading and would like to join a group of like-minded individuals on Facebook
HEALTHY BODY - HEALTHY MIND
at CommonSenseFactor.us

ABOUT THE AUTHOR

At the tender age of seven, a young boy felt the tremors of a changing world around him. His parents' divorce etched the first emotional scar on his heart. These early experiences trailed him, metamorphosing into anxiety and codependency that influenced many facets of his adulthood. Yet, rather than being chained to this narrative, Peter chose transformation.

His quest for healing took a pivotal turn in 2014 when he immersed himself in the world of hypnotherapy. Unraveling the mind's mysteries, he accessed and reframed the traumas nestled in its depths. By 2015, his journey expanded, understanding the interplay between mental and physical well-being, leading him to train as a health coach.

Amidst the chaos of the pandemic, while many felt the pressing weight of uncertainty, Peter's familiar foe – anxiety – once again made its presence felt. But this adversity birthed brilliance. He penned "*Got Smoothie Go – It's A Nutrient Rich Life – Your Smoothie Guide to Detox, Fighting Disease, Muscle Health, Healthy Weight Loss & Vibrant Living.*" This book was more than words on paper; it was the genesis of Common Sense Factor Book Publishing. A venture reflecting Peter's drive to sprinkle practical wisdom onto the canvas of life, providing tools for others as he once sought for himself.

Peter's introspective journey continued, resulting in "Courageous New Dawn: Mastering Your Mindset: Overcoming Fear, Conquering Anxiety, and Thriving in the Post-Pandemic World." But he didn't stop there. Drawing from his experiences, Peter presents another gem: "Courageous New Dawn: Healing Verses – Poetry Navigating Pain, Emotion, and Renewed Strength in 50+ Shades of Feelings." Through this collection, he seeks to tell every reader: In your battles, know you are not alone.

Peter's life is a testament to the values he holds dear, captured beautifully in the ethos of 'Common Sense Factor':

As you immerse yourself in Peter's writings, you're invited to read, feel, heal, and journey alongside a man who embodies resilience and empathy. Step into these pages, and perhaps you'll discover a reflection of your own story and the inspiration to continue your journey.

A note from the Author:

Readers might observe that the table of contents doesn't follow a traditional alphabetical format. This intentional design underscores the idea that emotions don't necessarily adhere to a chronological order. Depending on one's current emotions, one can select the relevant chapter. To assist in this, every poem's title incorporates the associated feeling to the best extent possible.

C - Compassionate
O - Optimistic
M - Mindful
M - Motivated
O - Observant
N - Nurturing

S - Sincere
E - Empathetic
N - Nonjudgmental
S - Self-aware
E - Ethical

F - Forward-thinking
A - Adaptable
C - Cognizant
T - Tolerant
O - Objective
R - Resilient

Visit The Author's Page at
AuthorEnd.com

CONTENTS

1. Fear and Anxiety Amise   1
2. Has the World Gone Mad?   3
3. Where Life Isn't So Common   5
4. For the Fearful Heart   7
5. Courageous New Dawn: A Nostalgic Verse   9
6. From Shadows to Dawn: The Liberation of Shame   11
7. Awakening of the Bold: A Dance with Confidence   13
8. Dusk's Promise: Embracing Tomorrow's Light   15
9. When Proudly We Stand   17
10. Embrace of the Dawn: Hope Beyond Sorrow   19
11. Amidst the Din: The Dawn of Inner Clarity   21
12. Phoenix Rise: Embracing the Dawn Amidst Despair   23
13. Embracing the Dawn: The Dance of Unexpected Turns   25
14. Embers of Hope: Navigating Life's Sudden Storm   27
15. Dawn's Promise: A Beacon Through Worried Nights   29
16. The Blush of Dawn: Rising Above Embarrassment   31
17. When Guilt Shadows the Heart   33
18. Whispers of Dawn: An Anthem for the Shy Soul   35
19. From Fury to Dawn: The Heart's Guided Light   37
20. Dawn's Symphony of Delight: An Ode to Joy   39
21. Whispers of the Courageous New Dawn   41
22. Embracing Solitude: Heralding the Courageous Dawn   43

23. Luminous Horizon: Navigating the Mind's Labyrinth — 45
24. Dawn's Promise: A Beacon Amidst the Overwhelm — 47
25. Embrace of the Dawn: Moments of Serenity — 49
26. When Anxiety Whispers, Dawn Speaks Louder — 51
27. Whispers of the Dawn: The Dance of Inspiration — 53
28. Rising Above: Strength in Humility's Shadow — 55
29. Release at Dawn: Transcending Resentment's Hold — 57
30. Annoyance's Echo: Lessons in the Dawn — 59
31. Emergence: From Overwhelm to Dawn — 61
32. Whispers of Wonder: Dawn's Curious Dance — 63
33. From Indifference to Dawn: A Journey Within — 65
34. Dawning Euphoria: The Pulse of New Beginnings — 67
35. Echoes of Empathy: The Dawn's Embrace — 69
36. Apathy's Dim, Courageous Dawn Shines — 71
37. Elation's Dawn: The Symphony of Renewal — 73
38. Dawning Relief: A Symphony of Renewed Hope — 75
39. Embracing Solitude: The Silver Lining of Loneliness — 77
40. Awakening in the Quiet: The Gift of Boredom — 79
41. Dawn's Quiet Symphony: The Dance of Contentment — 81
42. From Envy to Enlightenment: The Dawn's Lesson — 83
43. Emergence from Shadows: The Dawn of Shame-Free Being — 85
44. Unyielding Pride: Dawn's Resonance — 87
45. Emergence from Shadows: Dawn Over Despair — 89
46. Luminance of Hope: The Dawn's Eternal Song — 91

47. Dawn's Remedy: Beyond the Shadows of Doubt 93
48. Dawn's Trust: The Beacon of Hope 95
49. Awaiting the Dawn: The Pulse of Anticipation 97
50. Disgust's Dance: Deciphering the Hidden Song 99
51. Whispers of Wonder: The Dance of Dawn and Surprise 101
52. Dawn's Embrace: A Symphony of Gratitude 103
53. Emerald Insights: Lessons from Jealousy's Hold 105
54. Boundless Dawn: The Eternal Embrace of Love 107
55. Dance of Dawn: Embracing Fear's Guiding Light 109
56. Reference 112

1
FEAR AND ANXIETY AMISE

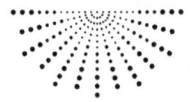

In a world once veiled in uncertain haze,

Where shadows of fear cast long, dark days,

Comes a beacon, a hope, a courageous new dawn,

Signaling to us all: It's time to move on.

In the still of the night, when anxieties stir,

Echoes of the past, a world that once was,

Rise above the whispers, the echoes of doubt,

Mastering mindset is what life's about.

Fear, a foe familiar, dressed in disguise,

Tells tales of despair beneath starry skies,

Yet within every heart, there lies a flame,

It is a power to overcome, to rewrite the game.

Conquer anxiety, that thief in the night,

With wisdom and courage, with innermost light,

For even in darkness, one truth remains clear,

The power to thrive is stronger than fear.

Post-pandemic memories, some bitter, some sweet,

Have taught us resilience and made us complete.

Embrace every lesson; let not one be in vain,

For through every storm, there's wisdom to gain.

Now, stand at the brink of a world reborn,

Embrace the challenges, the thorns and the thorn,

For with every sunrise, a promise is made,

Of a courageous new dawn, where hopes never fade.

Master your thoughts, let them dance, let them soar,

For in the heart of the brave, fear is no more.

Thriving and shining in a world so grand,

With the power of mindset, together we stand.

— P. LAST

2
HAS THE WORLD GONE MAD?

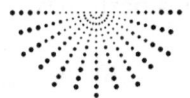

In a tempest of chaos, where reason seemed lost,

The world spun in madness, a tumultuous cost.

With every new headline, confusion spawned,

Yet from it emerged a courageous new dawn.

Amidst all the clamor, the shouts, and the cries,

A whisper emerged, cutting through the ties.

Seeking the truth in a world gone astray,

Courageous New Dawn would light up the way.

Has the world gone mad, or just unawakened?

To the heartbeats of hope, to the dreams left behind?

Yet from every corner, from darkness to light,

A spirit is rising, ready to fight.

Against the tide of despair, against the unknown,

For a world more compassionate, where love is shown.

Where even in madness, one can find a thread,

Of hope, of connection, a path to be led.

Courageous New Dawn, in this world so askew,

Offers a promise, a vision anew.

To navigate the chaos, to rise above the sad,

To find our way forward when the world's gone mad.

In the heart of the storm, where wild winds blow,

A seed of resilience continues to grow.

For even in madness, there's beauty to be had,

And it starts with the courage to ask,

"Has the world gone mad?"

— P. LAST

3
WHERE LIFE ISN'T SO COMMON

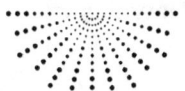

In a realm where the ordinary fades,

'Courageous New Dawn' lights uncharted shades.

Beyond the mundane, past familiar skies,

A journey to where true adventure lies.

Life isn't as common as most would deem,

When dreams blend with reality, and fantasy seems.

Awaken the spirit, let wonder take flight,

For in this new dawn, the stars shine so bright.

The footsteps we trace on this uncommon path,

Guide us away from routine's aftermath.

Where curiosity leads, and passions ignite,

In the embrace of a dawn, so courageously bright.

Venture into the unknown, where stories entwine,

Where limits are stretched and destinies align.

Seek the uncommon, let your spirit be free,

For 'Courageous New Dawn' is where you're meant to be.

Beyond horizons, where tales are reborn,

In the embrace of a day, unlike the foregone.

Celebrate the rare, the unique, and the known,

In this 'Courageous New Dawn,' life's beauty is shown.

— P. LAST

4
FOR THE FEARFUL HEART

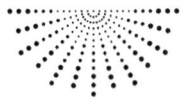

In the hushed whispers of the fearful night,

When shadows dance, stealing the moon's light,

Remember, there's a promise, a strength deep within,

A courageous new dawn where new days begin.

When the weight of the world seems too much to bear,

And the gusts of doubt pollute the air,

Know that within you, there's a fire that's true,

The flame of courage burning brightly in you.

Past traumas may haunt, like ghosts of old,

Their stories, like chains, are often retold,

But the power to break free, to rewrite your song,

Lies in your heart, where you've been strong all along.

Emotional triggers, like storms, may arise,

Darkening your skies, masking the prize,

But awaken the child, innocent and pure,

To lead you to harbors, safe and secure.

For fear is but a moment, a blink in time's vast span,

With courage as your compass, you'll rise, and you'll stand,

In the glow of a new dawn, where hope's light does weave,

A tapestry of strength for all who believe.

So, when afraid, remember this truth so profound,

With every courageous step, new horizons are found,

Embrace the journey, let fear fall apart,

For a courageous new dawn starts in the heart.

— P. LAST

5
COURAGEOUS NEW DAWN: A NOSTALGIC VERSE

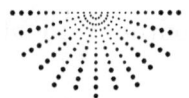

In the tender embrace of memories old,

Where the heart finds tales of yore retold,

There's a whispering wind, a gentle refrain,

Of days gone by, sunlit, washed by rain.

The innocence of laughter, the soft hum of a tune,

Golden summers that faded, winters' silver moon.

The dance of shadows, the play of the light,

In the warmth of yesterday, our souls took flight.

Yet amidst these moments, where time seems to pause,

Lies the strength of a dawn, a courageous cause.

For within every memory, in every silent tear,

Is a lesson, a promise, a hope crystal clear.

The child within us, with dreams ever vast,

Looks back to the past, yet is built to last.

In nostalgia's embrace, we find not just a trace,

But a fire, a passion, a quickening pace.

As we remember and journey through time,

We rise with resilience, mountains we climb.

A courageous new dawn, with each memory's gleam,

Guiding us forward while holding a dream.

So let nostalgia guide, with its soft, gentle hand,

To a future so bright, in a promising land.

For with every glance back, we gather the drive,

To awaken our spirits and truly thrive.

— P. LAST

6
FROM SHADOWS TO DAWN: THE LIBERATION OF SHAME

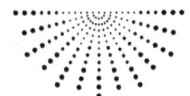

In the muted light of regrets past,

Where shadows of shame seem to hold us fast,

From the depth emerges a courageous new dawn,

Whispering gently, "It's time to move on."

Shame has a voice, cold and stern,

Echoing lessons we'd rather unlearn.

Yet, beneath the weight of the guilt we've known,

There's a resilience, silently grown.

For in every heart that has tasted despair,

A flicker remains a light that's rare.

Courageous New Dawn, guide us true,

To face our shame and emerge anew.

Acceptance is the bridge we must cross,

To heal the wounds, to mourn the loss.

For in embracing our flaws and our past,

We find strength unsurpassed.

In the embrace of the morning's first light,

Shame's heavy chains become feather-light.

With Courageous New Dawn leading the way,

We rise, unburdened, into a new day.

For every shame has a lesson to teach,

A destination, a dream to reach.

So, take the hand of the Courageous New Morn,

And know that from shame, strength is born.

— P. LAST

7
AWAKENING OF THE BOLD: A DANCE WITH CONFIDENCE

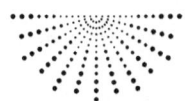

Amidst the mists of yesteryears gone by,

Where shadows and whispers did oft belie,

Emerges a spirit, bold and profound,

For within a confident heart, true strength is found.

No longer chained by the doubts of the past,

With 'Courageous New Dawn,' confidence is amassed,

The traumas that once pulled the spirit asunder,

Now, fuel the fire of passion and wonder.

With every step of this enlightening spree,

Discover the power of the confident 'me,'

For within these pages, the secrets unfold,

Of how to be fearless, audacious, and bold.

The inner child laughs, free from its cage,

Dancing with joy, transcending its age,

Gone are the triggers, the hurts, and the scorn,

In this 'Courageous New Dawn,' a confident self is reborn.

So, arise with aplomb, let your spirit dive deep,

Harness your power, awaken from sleep,

With confidence glowing like the first morning light,

Embrace your 'Courageous New Dawn,' and take flight.

— P. LAST

8
DUSK'S PROMISE: EMBRACING TOMORROW'S LIGHT

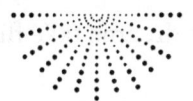

In the hush of twilight, when the world seems dim,

When strength feels scant and hopes grow slim,

When weariness blankets like dusk's quiet sprawl,

Remember the call of the Courageous New Dawn.

When feet tread heavy and dreams feel far,

When shadows of doubt bear each falling star,

Take heart in the promise, though the night be long,

For there lies the whisper of a dawn's new song.

Rest, dear traveler, but do not despair,

For within every dusk, dawn waits to bear,

A new day, a new strength, a zest to belong,

To the embrace of the light where the brave grow strong.

Exhaustion is a teacher, not just a phase,

In its silent depths, wisdom stays,

For even in weariness, a truth does spawn,

After the night comes a Courageous New Dawn.

So rest and recover, let dreams take flight,

In the gentle embrace of the starlit night,

For with the morning, you'll rise, reborn,

Champion of challenges in the Courageous New Dawn.

— P. LAST

9
WHEN PROUDLY WE STAND

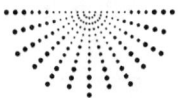

In the heart of the morning, as daybreak unveils,

Where hope and horizon, where strength never fails,

In that luminous moment, when shadows withdraw,

Courageous New Dawn is the pride that we saw.

From memories past, where our battles were fought,

To the promise of futures, by bravery sought,

In every endeavor, in each challenge faced,

There's a dawn we create and a pride embraced.

For those moments of triumph, when barriers fall,

When we rise from our knees, standing tall, standing all,

When voices of doubt are silenced and gone,

It's the pride of the journey, the song we've drawn.

In the echoes of victories, in tales often spun,

It's not just the battles but how they were won,

With heart and with spirit, with passion and grit,

For the Courageous New Dawn, in pride, we commit.

So here in this instant, as gratitude beams,

For every hurdle surpassed, for every dream,

Let's raise a toast to the path we're upon,

For the Courageous New Dawn and the pride that's drawn.

— P. LAST

10
EMBRACE OF THE DAWN: HOPE BEYOND SORROW

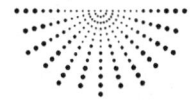

In the hush of the night, when tears softly fall,

And the weight of the world makes you feel oh so small,

Remember the promise of the Courageous New Dawn,

Whispering to your heart: "Dear soul, carry on."

When sadness engulfs like a stormy gray cloud,

And the cacophony of doubts seems unbearably loud,

Seek solace in the tales of hope and rebirth,

For every dusk has its purpose, as does every hurt.

Embrace the sorrows, for they're part of the tale,

Every ship, even strong ones, at times will face gale.

But with every tear shed, a lesson is revealed,

The strength to rise, a spirit unsealed.

Awaken the child that slumbers within,

The one full of wonder, who knew how to begin,

Rediscover their laughter, their joy, and their play,

For in their pure wisdom, the blues fade away.

The Courageous New Dawn beckons, gentle and true,

A beacon of hope, especially for you.

For even in sadness, in the heart's darkest dive,

There lies the power to rise, to thrive.

So, when you're feeling low, with spirits forlorn,

Remember the promise of the Courageous New Dawn.

In the embrace of its warmth, your sadness will wane,

Bringing new hope, strength, and an end to the pain.

— P. LAST

11
AMIDST THE DIN: THE DAWN OF INNER CLARITY

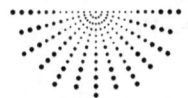

In a world swirling with ceaseless sound,

Where distractions reign, and thoughts abound,

A call to the soul, a whisper so slight,

Guides us toward the Courageous New Light.

When screens flicker, and sirens blare,

In a cacophony of chaos, it's hard to stare,

At the heart's true path, the purpose within,

Yet amidst the noise, our journey begins.

Distracted, we wander but not forever lost,

For in every moment, there's a hidden cost,

To be paid in attention, in focus, in time,

And the price of distraction? A mountain to climb.

But fear not the ascent, for with every stride,

The Courageous New Dawn waits, arms open wide,

To embrace the distracted, the weary, the worn,

And ignite in their hearts a new day reborn.

For distractions may challenge, may pull, may sway,

Yet the power to overcome is just a breath away.

In the quiet space between heartbeats, we find,

The Courageous New Dawn, a peace of the mind.

So when the world tugs and your thoughts go astray,

Remember the dawn and the promise of day.

For even amidst chaos, one truth remains tight,

With courage and focus, we conquer the night.

— P. LAST

12
PHOENIX RISE: EMBRACING THE DAWN AMIDST DESPAIR

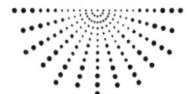

Amid a storm, when the winds loudly call,

When your feet stumble and shadows seem tall,

There's a whisper of hope, a courageous new light,

Guiding you through, turning day from the night.

Frustration's a fire, burning fierce and deep,

Challenging dreams, stirring emotions that weep.

But within every heart, beneath layers of pain,

Lies the strength of a dawn, waiting to reign.

Face that frustration, let its flames rise,

Yet, know it's a phoenix in clever disguise.

From these ashes of turmoil, of anger, of scorn,

A courageous spirit is reborn.

For every setback, every tear that might fall,

"Courageous New Dawn" stands tall through it all.

Offering solace, a hand to uplift,

Turning frustration into a powerful gift.

So, when walls seem unyielding and paths winding long,

Recall this anthem, your empowering song.

For in the dance of emotions, in the ebb and the dive,

"A Courageous New Dawn" helps you thrive.

— P. LAST

13
EMBRACING THE DAWN: THE DANCE OF UNEXPECTED TURNS

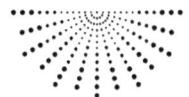

In the quiet lull of an unsuspected morn,

Where dreams seem distant and yet unborn,

There comes a gust, a swift turn of the tide,

A Courageous New Dawn, with arms opened wide.

Surprise in its essence, like dawn's early light,

Breaks through the veil of the darkest night.

It challenges notions, it alters our view,

Whispers of wonders, both old and new.

In every murmur of the unexpected,

There lies a lesson, a path redirected.

For in the surprise, be it joy or dismay,

A Courageous New Dawn beckons, leading the way.

With eyes wide open, in pure childlike glee,

We face the unknown; let our spirits run free.

For the heart that embraces change with a song,

Finds strength in the journey and becomes ever strong.

So let the winds of surprise sweep you along,

Find beauty in detours where you thought you belonged.

For each turn and twist in this dance, we call life,

Brings a Courageous New Dawn, cutting through strife.

— P. LAST

14
EMBERS OF HOPE: NAVIGATING LIFE'S SUDDEN STORM

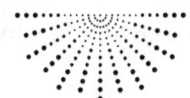

In a moment's stillness, when the world feels askew,

When the shock of the unseen casts a pallor hue,

Amidst the trembles and the heart's silent cry,

Courageous New Dawn whispers, urging you to try.

For shock is but a moment, a pause in life's dance,

A reminder of frailty, of fate's vast expanse.

Yet, within the sudden gasps of disbelief,

There's a strength that emerges, a profound relief.

A new dawn awaits, bold and unafraid,

Offering a hand, a promise un-swayed.

For every heartache and every dismay,

Courageous New Dawn lights a brighter way.

Shock may cloud vision, may tether the soul,

But like the sun after rain, there's a brighter role.

In the heart of the tempest, the storm's wild churn,

There's a lesson, a message, an opportunity to learn.

So, amidst the chaos, when you feel lost and spun,

Know that a new dawn, a courageous one, has begun.

Hold onto hope, let it be your guide,

For even in shock, courage resides inside.

— P. LAST

15
DAWN'S PROMISE: A BEACON THROUGH WORRIED NIGHTS

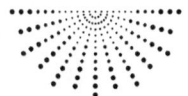

In the vast realm of thoughts, where worries weave,

Where doubt and fear interlace, deceive,

There's a horizon, radiant and true,

The Courageous New Dawn beckons to you.

When the night is thick, and stars seem dim,

And the weight of the world pulls at your brim,

Lift your eyes, see the dawn's early light,

A beacon, a promise, cutting through night.

For every moment of worry and woe,

There's a lesson, a strength yet to show,

In the heart of the storm, amidst thunder's song,

Know that with courage, you can't go wrong.

The whispers of anxiety, the shadows of fear,

Are mere fleeting clouds as dawn draws near.

Embrace the morning, its golden embrace,

For in its light, worries find no place.

So whenever you're lost, feeling adrift in the night,

Turn to the Courageous New Dawn, your beacon of light.

With hope as your compass and strength as your guide,

Beyond every worry, bright horizons reside.

— P. LAST

16
THE BLUSH OF DAWN: RISING ABOVE EMBARRASSMENT

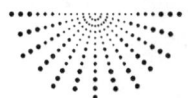

In the hush of twilight, a blush does appear,

A moment's unease, the feeling so clear.

Embarrassment's touch, a temporary sting,

But in the Courageous New Dawn, it's a fleeting thing.

For each red-faced instance, a lesson to learn,

Not a mark of failure but a chance to discern.

Though the cheeks might heat, and the heart might race,

In this newfound light, we find our true place.

In the vast cosmic dance, where stars freely fall,

Mistakes are but steps, a part of it all.

Each stumble or misstep, each blush or dismay,

Is a part of the journey, the price that we pay.

But Courageous New Dawn brings a promise so true,

That embarrassment's grip won't linger or rue.

Instead, with each blush, with each falter or slip,

We're taught to rise up, to regain our grip.

To embrace every flaw, every error, each scar,

For they make us human; they make us who we are.

And in the gentle embrace of the Courageous New Morn,

Even embarrassment feels newly reborn.

For it's not about hiding or masking the pain,

But understanding it, taming it, breaking its chain.

In the glow of the Dawn, where courage does gleam,

Even our weakest moments can be turned into dreams.

— P. LAST

17
WHEN GUILT SHADOWS THE HEART

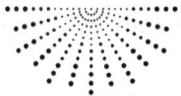

In the silent chambers of remorseful minds,

Where guilt weaves tales of mistakes left behind,

There rises a call, both gentle and firm,

A voice from the heart, where all truths belong.

Courageous New Dawn, shine your light on me,

Dispel these dark clouds, set my conscience free.

For in the weight of regret, my spirit feels bound,

Yet, with hope and with grace, redemption is found.

Each step that I took, each choice that I made,

Has etched a story in memories displayed.

But mistakes are but lessons in life's grand design,

And the power to change is, and always, mine.

Embrace me, O Dawn, with your forgiving hue,

Teach me to forgive myself and others, too.

For guilt is but a moment, a transient phase,

And with courage, I'll rise, leaving behind guilt's maze.

So when shadows grow long, and night seems to stay,

Let the Courageous New Dawn light the way.

In its embrace, may guilt's weight be withdrawn,

For a brighter tomorrow, in a new light reborn.

— P. LAST

18
WHISPERS OF DAWN: AN ANTHEM FOR THE SHY SOUL

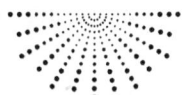

In the quiet corners of the world, where whispers tread,

Where thoughts swirl silently inside a cautious head,

There blooms a tale, an anthem, a song so uniquely spun,

Of a Courageous New Dawn waiting for everyone.

Feeling shy is but a cloud, a misty veil to see,

A delicate embrace of what used to be.

Yet beneath that timid shade, a strength does reside,

A dormant force, a passion too powerful to hide.

Each hesitant heartbeat, each fleeting glance away,

Holds stories of dreams, waiting for their day.

But with the dawn comes a courage to speak what's in your core,

To share the beauty inside, to let your spirit soar.

For in the gentle spaces between each quiet word,

The voice of the shy begs to be heard.

"Courageous New Dawn," calls out to thee,

"Awaken the brave; let your spirit roam free."

So when shadows of shyness cloud the path you're on,

Remember the power of a new dawn song.

For even in silence, in moments withdrawn,

Lies the courage to rise, to greet the dawn.

— P. LAST

19
FROM FURY TO DAWN: THE HEART'S GUIDED LIGHT

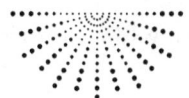

In the heart's emotional furnace, where anger ignites,

Where feelings flare up, and the spirit alights,

Remember, dear soul, in the heat of the fray,

A courageous new dawn is just a breath away.

When tempests of fury cloud judgment and sight,

And the world feels awry, and nothing seems right,

Seek solace in stillness, let your heartstrings play,

A harmonious tune of a brighter new day.

The fire of anger, unbridled, unchecked,

Can ravage the spirit, leaving souls wrecked.

But harness that power, let it lead the way,

To lessons learned and a wiser foray.

For within every rage, there's a cry to be heard,

A voice of the wounded, a soul that's been stirred.

Listen, embrace, understand, and then see,

The path to healing, to being set free.

Courageous New Dawn, when emotions run high,

Guides you to face them, to reach for the sky.

For anger, though fierce, can illuminate too,

The shadows and corners we need to look through.

So when fury engulfs, and the heart feels the strain,

Remember the promise of hope's gentle rain.

For with every sunset, that anger might spawn,

There's the promise of peace in a Courageous New Dawn.

— P. LAST

20
DAWN'S SYMPHONY OF DELIGHT: AN ODE TO JOY

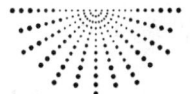

In the heart's radiant expanse where laughter does play,

There's a dance of delight in the light of the day,

Where the winds of joy whisper tales of yore,

There, the 'Courageous New Dawn' begins to explore.

Golden beams of happiness cascade from the sky,

As dreams take wing, and spirits fly high.

In every chuckle, in every cheerful song,

There's a power that tells us to joy we belong.

Awaken, dear heart, let happiness flow,

For in the realms of joy, radiant colors do grow.

Every moment of glee, every beat of elation,

Guides us to a dawn of jubilant celebration.

The world seems brighter, the flowers more fair,

When happiness echoes in the free, open air.

With 'Courageous New Dawn,' embrace the glee,

For in joy's embrace, our souls dance free.

So when the skies are blue, and your spirit feels light,

Turn to this anthem, shining so bright.

For with each happy note, with each jubilant tide,

'Courageous New Dawn' is forever by your side.

— P. LAST

21
WHISPERS OF THE COURAGEOUS NEW DAWN

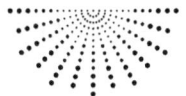

In the muted moments, when nerves do fray,

When shadows lengthen, stealing light away,

Hear the whispers of a Courageous New Dawn,

Telling you boldly, "Carry on, carry on."

When your heart flutters, like a caged bird's wing,

And trepidation makes it hard to sing,

Recall the promise, the strength you've drawn,

From every challenge, every dusk till dawn.

For nerves are but ripples on a vast, vast sea,

Temporary and fleeting, like the wind in a tree.

Yet deep within, where your true self does reside,

Is a dawn of courage, impossible to hide.

Embrace the tremble, let it be your guide,

To realms of growth, where fears subside.

For in facing the nerves, in dancing with doubt,

The Courageous New Dawn within bursts out.

So when you're feeling nervous, in the night's embrace,

Think of the dawn, its gentle grace.

And let its courage fill you, let its light be shown,

For with every new dawn, see how you've grown.

— P. LAST

22
EMBRACING SOLITUDE: HERALDING THE COURAGEOUS DAWN

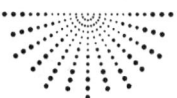

In the silent moments, when loneliness creeps,

When the world feels vast and one's spirit weeps,

Remember the promise of the Courageous New Dawn,

Whispering softly, "With strength, carry on."

When solitude's weight bears heavy on the chest,

And it feels like the heart has taken a rest,

In the quiet, a gentle reminder is drawn,

There's warmth in the glow of the Courageous New Dawn.

For even in isolation, shadows, and doubt,

There's a fire within, waiting to sprout.

Though alone you might feel, in the vastness of night,

The dawn offers solace, a comforting light.

Embrace the journey, let loneliness be,

A catalyst for growth, setting the spirit free.

With each lonely tear, resilience is born,

In the embrace of the Courageous New Dawn.

Remember, you're never as alone as you seem,

With dreams to be dreamt and visions to dream.

For in solitude's depth, a truth is redrawn,

You're held and uplifted by the Courageous New Dawn.

— P. LAST

23
LUMINOUS HORIZON: NAVIGATING THE MIND'S LABYRINTH

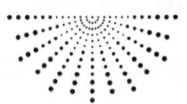

In the maze of thoughts where confusion does thread,

Where clarity's fogged, and certainties shed,

In that twilight space, where doubts do spawn,

Shines the guiding light of Courageous New Dawn.

When pathways entangle, and choices run vast,

And the voices of yesterday echo the past,

Hold tight to your compass, though vision be gone,

For its needle points to Courageous New Dawn.

The fog may be thick, the journey unclear,

But embrace every moment and let go of the fear.

For in heart's quiet whisper, the truth is drawn,

Guiding souls to the embrace of Courageous New Dawn.

Remember the strength that within you resides,

When confusion's web, your spirit derides.

With patience and faith, darkness is withdrawn,

Revealing the horizon of Courageous New Dawn.

So, when the world blurs and paths intertwine,

Trust in your journey; let your heart be the sign.

For even in chaos, hope is brightly drawn,

In the comforting glow of Courageous New Dawn.

— P. LAST

24
DAWN'S PROMISE: A BEACON AMIDST THE OVERWHELM

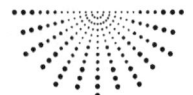

In the rush of the tide, when waves crest high,

And the world seems vast beneath the sprawling sky,

Remember, there's a dawn, courageous and true,

Waiting on the horizon, waiting for you.

When burdens amass, and the shadows creep in,

When the clamor grows loud, drowning out your own din,

Seek solace in the promise of a brighter new morn,

For in "Courageous New Dawn", hope is reborn.

The weight of the world may press on your heart,

Chaos swirling around, pulling you apart,

But within these pages, find solace and guide,

A beacon to light up the turbulent ride.

Embrace the journey, with its twists and turns,

For every challenge faced, a brighter fire burn,

With each step forward, with each rising sun,

Know that battles, though fierce, can indeed be won.

So when you're feeling lost, adrift in the night,

Hold tight to the promise of dawn's breaking light,

For in the embrace of "Courageous New Dawn,"

The strength to persevere is drawn upon.

— P. LAST

25
EMBRACE OF THE DAWN: MOMENTS OF SERENITY

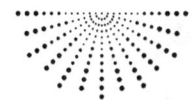

In the silent embrace of morning's first light,

When the world's still asleep and the stars take their flight,

There's a moment, a whisper, a hush that is drawn,

A feeling of serenity with Courageous New Dawn.

The waters lie still, reflecting the sky,

As traumas and fears are left far behind.

Emotions once raging, now calmly respond,

To the gentle caress of Courageous New Dawn.

The inner child laughs, free and unbound,

As peace and tranquility all around are found.

The triggers and tempests, once fierce, are now gone,

Swept away by the breeze of Courageous New Dawn.

With each breath we take, serenity grows,

A balm for old wounds, a salve for our woes.

For in this new day, a promise is drawn,

Of hope, love, and healing in Courageous New Dawn.

So when your heart seeks a haven so rare,

Find solace in moments when dawn meets the air.

Let serenity guide you; let it be drawn,

Into the embrace of Courageous New Dawn.

— P. LAST

26
WHEN ANXIETY WHISPERS, DAWN SPEAKS LOUDER

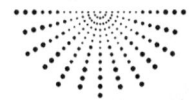

In the hushed grip of anxiety's clutch,

When the world feels too heavy, too much,

There's a light, a beacon, a soft, distant call,

Of the Courageous New Dawn, awaiting us all.

When your breath comes in short and shadows grow long,

And the melody falters in life's ongoing song,

Remember, there's strength in the tales we've spun,

In the heart of the storm, we become one.

Breathe in the promise of a brand-new day,

Where fear's fleeting whispers are kept at bay.

For even in moments of tremulous fright,

The dawn promises solace, bringing new light.

Hold close to your heart the innate hope,

With every heartbeat, it's never too late.

To rise, to conquer, to stand up and say,

"I've faced my anxieties and cast them away."

So when you're ensnared in doubt's chilling dance,

Think of the Courageous New Dawn's radiant glance.

For in its embrace, you're never alone,

Guided by love to a peace yet unknown.

— P. LAST

27
WHISPERS OF THE DAWN: THE DANCE OF INSPIRATION

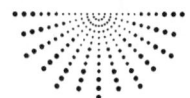

In the gentle whispers of the morn,

When dreams are born, and hopes are worn,

There lies a tale, a song, a call,

Of the Courageous New Dawn for all.

Lift your eyes to the horizon wide,

Where inspiration dances side by side,

With dreams that sparkle, passions that glow,

And the courage to chase where wild winds blow.

Each heartbeat, a rhythm, a resonant song,

Pushing us forward, making us strong,

For within our spirit, fierce and profound,

It is the spark of a dawn, unceasing, unbound.

The canvas of life, vast and untamed,

Calls out to the brave, the wild, the unnamed,

To paint with bold strokes, with love and elation,

A world shaped by pure inspiration.

For every challenge, every trial we face,

There's a moment of magic, a saving grace,

In the Courageous New Dawn, bright and true,

Where inspiration is reborn, and dreams come through.

So when darkness looms and hopes seem slight,

Remember the dawn, its radiant light,

For within its embrace, every fear will wane,

And inspiration will guide us time and again.

— P. LAST

28
RISING ABOVE: STRENGTH IN HUMILITY'S SHADOW

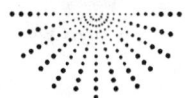

In the hush of the dusk, when shadows grow long,

When the world seems to echo a mockingbird's song,

When the weight of humiliation feels too vast,

Remember, these moments, they too shall pass.

For in the annals of time, it's but a brief spell,

A fleeting whisper, a transient swell.

Courageous New Dawn, rise up from the plight,

Turn the tide of the darkness and embrace the first light.

Your worth isn't bound by the laughter of foes,

Nor is it tethered where the cold wind blows.

True value's intrinsic, deep within the soul,

Not judged by the moments you weren't in control.

With every sun that sets, a new day is born,

A chance to rewrite, to wear a new thorn.

Face the sting of the past but with a steadfast gaze,

See a future unburdened, free of old haze.

So when you stumble, when you feel small,

When humiliation makes you feel two feet tall,

Think of the Courageous New Dawn, waiting ahead,

Where humility's power replaces dread.

For in the dance of life, twirls will confound,

But with inner courage, true strength is found.

Reclaim your story, wear your scars with pride,

For with every fall, there's a rise worldwide.

— P. LAST

29
RELEASE AT DAWN: TRANSCENDING RESENTMENT'S HOLD

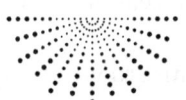

In the quiet corners of hearts, resentment grew,

A silent storm, darkening the sky's pure hue,

But with each brave step on this dawn's golden path,

We learn to release, to free our soul's wrath.

Courageous New Dawn, where healing begins,

Challenging the shadows, the root of our sins,

Resentment, a chain binding us tight,

Yet dawn promises freedom, a radiant light.

The weight of the past, heavy and stark,

Yet in every heartbeat, there lies a spark,

A call to forgiveness, to understanding true,

For resentment harms the holder more than it's due.

In the embrace of dawn, where courage does lie,

Resentment finds its release with a heartfelt sigh,

For in the light of understanding, shadows fade away,

And the heart finds peace in the light of the day.

Courageous New Dawn teaches us to see,

Beyond the chains of hurt to what we can be,

Free from resentment, awakened and alive,

In the heart of the dawn, we truly thrive.

— P. LAST

30
ANNOYANCE'S ECHO: LESSONS IN THE DAWN

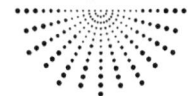

In the dawning light of a brand-new day,

Where hope and courage come out to play,

There still lingers, like a pesky fly,

The niggling feeling we can't deny.

Annoyance, a thorn in the foot of our stride,

A whispering wind against the tide.

Yet, in this Courageous New Dawn we see,

Even annoyance has its decree.

It teaches us patience, asks us to pause,

Reflect on the root, the underlying cause.

Is it a memory, a past trauma's sting?

Or an echo of the hurt life can sometimes bring?

But the dawn is resilient, and so are we,

Turning annoyance into opportunity.

For every irritation, every little poke,

It is a chance to heal, to rise, to evoke.

In the vast spectrum of emotions so wide,

Annoyance, too, has its rightful side.

In this Courageous New Dawn, we're spun,

Every feeling has its place under the sun.

So when annoyance comes knocking at your door,

Acknowledge, reflect, and dive into its core.

For in this journey of growth and rebirth,

Every emotion has its worth.

— P. LAST

31
EMERGENCE: FROM OVERWHELM TO DAWN

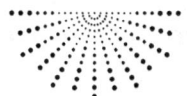

In the heart of the tempest, where feelings cascade,

Overwhelm takes the stage, casting shadows and shade.

A tidal wave of thoughts and emotions run deep,

Drowning out clarity, stealing sleep.

But within the maelstrom, a dawn does await,

Courageous and steadfast, it's never too late.

To harness the storm, to stand tall and firm,

To find the eye's calm, to take a new term.

For every emotion, intense and profound,

Carries a lesson, a message unbound.

In the grip of overwhelm, when clarity's gone,

There's strength in the struggle, a new day to dawn.

Embrace the turbulence, let it refine,

Like a diamond from coal, let your spirit shine.

For after the storm, with its fury and might,

Comes a courageous new dawn, bathed in soft light.

Overwhelm is a moment, a chapter, a phase,

But with courage and hope, we can set our own ways.

In the heart of the storm, let this truth be your song,

With a courageous new dawn, we emerge strong.

— P. LAST

32
WHISPERS OF WONDER: DAWN'S CURIOUS DANCE

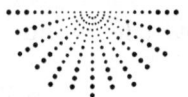

In the heart of the morning, where new dreams are born,

There's a whisper of wonder, a courageous new dawn.

Curiosity beckons like the first light of day,

Guiding us forward, showing the way.

With every question, there's a story to tell,

A journey through valleys, over mountains as well.

The world spins a mystery, vast and profound,

In 'Courageous New Dawn,' the answers are found.

What lies in the shadows? What dreams may come true?

Curiosity's dance is ever so new.

Awaken the child, whose eyes gleam so wide,

At the marvels and mysteries life does provide.

The world is a canvas, so vast and so deep,

With secrets, it whispers and promises it keeps.

Yet in this brave dawning, when all feels so new,

Curiosity's fire will carry us through.

So embrace the unknown, let wonder take flight,

In the heart of the dawn, in the soft morning light.

For with every question, the universe spawns,

A tale of discovery in the 'Courageous New Dawn.'

— P. LAST

33
FROM INDIFFERENCE TO DAWN: A JOURNEY WITHIN

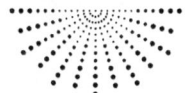

In the vast expanse of emotions, we span,

Indifference stands, a silent, still man.

Not a ripple of joy nor a tremor of fear,

Its voice is a whisper, often too faint to hear.

Yet amidst the colors of feelings so bright,

Indifference exists, like day turning to night.

It's neither the dark nor the radiant morn,

But the space in-between, where the wearied are born.

Courageous New Dawn, with promise anew,

Calls out to this void with a perspective so true.

For indifference, though still, has a story to tell,

Of moments missed and dreams that fell.

But as day breaks and the sun begins to climb,

The indifferent heart can, too, change with time.

For buried beneath that indifferent shroud,

Lies a spark waiting, quiet yet loud.

The Courageous New Dawn whispers, "Awake, arise,"

Turn indifference to action; open those eyes.

For even in stillness, a purpose is found,

In the Courageous New Dawn, let your passion resound.

— P. LAST

34
DAWNING EUPHORIA: THE PULSE OF NEW BEGINNINGS

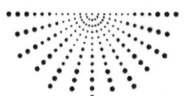

In the heart of the horizon, where the new day is drawn,

There pulses a beat, the rhythm of a song.

A melody of hope, of dreams yet to spawn,

That's the thrill, the excitement of Courageous New Dawn.

With every fresh step, where past shadows once lay,

Comes a dance of delight, a brilliant display.

The thrill of the unknown, the joy of what's gone,

Ignites the soul's fire, as we're drawn to press on.

The winds carry whispers of adventures to come,

Of battles, we'll win and victories to be won.

The heart races faster to a future redrawn,

In the brilliant, breathtaking, Courageous New Dawn.

The world is alive, with possibilities vast,

With each moment, a bridge to the future from the past.

Excitement's the beacon, leading us on and on,

To the luminous horizons of Courageous New Dawn.

So embrace the elation; let it be your guide,

Through challenges, fears, and life's roller-coaster ride.

For in every beat, in every new drawn yawn,

There's the zest, the zeal, of Courageous New Dawn.

— P. LAST

35
ECHOES OF EMPATHY: THE DAWN'S EMBRACE

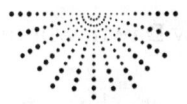

In the heart of the morning, where whispers begin,

There's a sentiment deep, a feeling within.

It's more than just seeing or hearing a cry,

It's feeling the depth of the soul's silent sigh.

In the vastness of pain or the glisten of joy,

Empathy reaches out, a bridge to deploy.

For in the echo of heartbeats, in laughter or tears,

Courageous New Dawn makes one thing clear:

That to understand another, to truly perceive,

It is to walk in their shoes, to hope and believe.

In the soft-spoken tales of struggles and dreams,

Empathy listens in gentle moonbeams.

The world spins and turns, emotions ride high,

Yet, in the midst of it all, Empathy's nigh.

With open arms and a heart ready to feel,

It mends broken spirits; it helps wounds to heal.

For in Courageous New Dawn, where souls intertwine,

Empathy shines brightest, a beacon, a sign.

That we're never alone in sorrow or joy,

Together, we rise, redefining our worth.

— P. LAST

36
APATHY'S DIM, COURAGEOUS DAWN SHINES

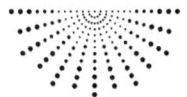

In a world painted grey, where feelings are scant,

Where passions fade away, and dreams feel distant and scant,

There's a silent battle with a ghost named Apathy,

A challenge not loud but silent, binding like gravity.

Yet, from this muted abyss, a whisper does call,

The "Courageous New Dawn" is a beacon for all.

For even in numbness, where emotions feel drawn,

There's a light that persists, a dawn to spawn.

Apathy's cloak, heavy and cold,

Hides vibrant colors, stories untold.

But every heart has a fire, a spark deep within,

Awaiting the moment for its revival to begin.

The journey isn't loud, no mountains to climb,

But a subtle step forward, taking one moment at a time.

Awakening the senses, the joy and the pain,

Embracing life's spectrum, feeling the sun and the rain.

So, in the land where feelings might stall,

Remember the call of the "Courageous New Dawn" tall.

For beyond the grey, beyond the night's yawn,

There's a world alive and vibrant, waiting to be drawn.

— P. LAST

37
ELATION'S DAWN: THE SYMPHONY OF RENEWAL

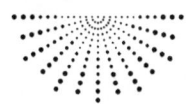

In the heart of the night, a spark ignites,

A sensation, a pulse, a dance of pure light.

Elation emerges, breaking the chains,

Bathing the soul, washing away pains.

From the depths of despair to the peaks so high,

Courageous New Dawn paints the sky.

Every hue of joy, every tint of delight,

Elation's song soars, taking its flight.

The shackles of yesteryears fall away,

As the dawn promises a brighter day.

The heart, once heavy, now light as a feather,

For the spirit knows no bounds, no tether.

In this radiant rise, we find our elation,

A symphony of hope, a soul's jubilation.

For in the embrace of Courageous New Dawn,

Elation is the anthem, and life sings on.

— P. LAST

38
DAWNING RELIEF: A SYMPHONY OF RENEWED HOPE

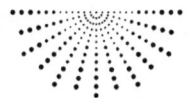

In the hush of twilight, when shadows wane,

And the weight of the past causes lingering pain,

There emerges a feeling, gentle and profound,

The soothing embrace of relief, unbound.

From the heart's deep caverns where worries reside,

To the mind's winding labyrinths where fears do hide,

Courageous New Dawn breaks, dispelling the night,

With a promise of hope, bathing all in its light.

Oh, the solace it brings, like a cool, gentle stream,

Washing away traumas like a forgotten dream.

Embracing the moments when the heart feels light,

As the shackles of yesteryears take their last flight.

For in this new dawning, where courage takes hold,

Relief is the story, beautifully told.

A narrative of freedom, of finding one's way,

In the vast, open horizons of a brand-new day.

So, breathe in the freshness, let go of the strife,

For relief is the dawn of a rejuvenated life.

In the heart of the brave, where new hopes are spun,

There's solace and peace with each rising sun.

— P. LAST

39
EMBRACING SOLITUDE: THE SILVER LINING OF LONELINESS

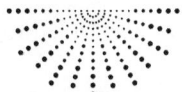

In the hush of the night, when the world feels so vast,

And the weight of the silence makes hearts beat so fast,

There's a cry deep within, a shadow of blue,

Loneliness whispers and the world feels askew.

But in this quiet realm, 'neath the vast starry dome,

Courageous New Dawn whispers softly, "You're not alone."

For in the depth of the void, in the vastness of night,

There's a spark, a connection, an ember so bright.

Loneliness, a journey, a pathway, a phase,

Can be filled with discovery, wonder, and praise.

For amidst the solitude, a truth does unfold,

That the heart, when it's open, is braver than bold.

The sun may retreat, and the world may seem bare,

But always remember, there's love in the air.

And as dawn breaks anew, with its promise so true,

Remember that loneliness is part of life's hue.

With Courageous New Dawn, let loneliness be,

A moment to reflect, to dream, and to see,

That even in silence, in the absence of song,

There's strength there's growth, and a place you belong.

— P. LAST

40
AWAKENING IN THE QUIET: THE GIFT OF BOREDOM

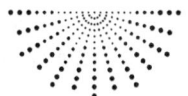

In the stillness of a moment when the world feels stark and bare,

When monotony's gray fingers weave a tapestry of despair,

In that silent, stretching chasm, where the soul feels all alone,

Comes a whisper of a challenge, a chance to truly hone.

For within the heart of boredom, where the colors seem to fade,

Lies the canvas of potential, waiting for its shade.

It's an invitation to explore and to create,

To ignite the inner passions, to redefine one's fate.

Courageous New Dawn beckons, with a promise pure and true,

Turn boredom into wonder, see the world with a fresher hue.

Awaken dreams dormant, let imagination run wild,

Discover the joy of a curious, ever-wandering child.

In the lull of the mundane, find a rhythm, find a rhyme,

For even in the quiet, there's a dance, a chime.

Embrace the silent moments, let them be a guide,

To a world of endless wonder, just waiting inside.

So when boredom comes knocking, see it not as a closed door,

But an opportunity waiting, a chance to explore.

With the heart of a savior, light the way so clear,

Turn boredom into beauty, and watch as wonders appear.

— P. LAST

41
DAWN'S QUIET SYMPHONY: THE DANCE OF CONTENTMENT

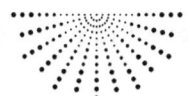

In the embrace of a gentle morn,

Where hopes and dreams are freshly born,

Lies the feeling, subtle and profound,

Of contentment, where peace is found.

In the midst of life's turbulent sea,

'Courageous New Dawn' teaches thee,

To find that harbor, that quiet space,

Where the heart beats at a tranquil pace.

The past may echo, shadows might play,

Yet, in this moment, all drifts away.

For contentment is a golden thread,

Weaving stories, both future and dead.

Awaken the child, that spirit free,

Dancing in joy beneath the old tree.

Conquering traumas, mastering fears,

Smiling in content, drying the tears.

For in this dawn, so brave and so new,

Contentment's song sings clear and true.

Rising, thriving, with each new day's light,

In the heart's content, we find our true might.

— P. LAST

42
FROM ENVY TO ENLIGHTENMENT: THE DAWN'S LESSON

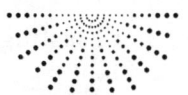

In the garden of feelings, envy grew wild,

Its venomous tendrils slyly beguiled.

Yet, in the heart of the Courageous New Dawn,

Lies strength to confront it, to draw upon.

Green-eyed monster, shadowing light's embrace,

Casting its doubts, trying to outpace,

But amidst the morning's radiant glow,

There's a lesson about envy we ought to know.

For it's not in what others may have or hold,

But the stories within us are untold and bold.

In the Courageous New Dawn, envy's just a phase,

A fleeting emotion in life's vast maze.

Instead of looking with longing at another's gain,

Find the treasures within and break envy's chain.

For in the brilliance of a new day's light,

Our true worth emerges gleaming and bright.

So, let envy be a teacher, not a lasting foe,

A reminder to nurture our own inner glow.

In the embrace of the Courageous New Dawn's might,

Transform envy into inspiration, and set your soul alight.

— P. LAST

43
EMERGENCE FROM SHADOWS: THE DAWN OF SHAME-FREE BEING

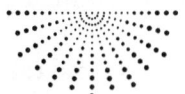

In the quiet corners of the heart's dim room,

Lies the heavy cloak of Shame, an all-encompassing gloom.

Yet, within the folds of such deep despair,

Courageous New Dawn whispers, "Venture if you dare."

For Shame, though powerful, is but a fleeting shade,

A construct of our fears in life's grand parade.

Yet, when we confront it in the light of dawn,

Its mighty façade crumbles, its strength withdrawn.

The sun of self-acceptance rises bold and true,

Illuminating darkness, casting a radiant hue.

No longer shackled, no longer confined,

In Courageous New Dawn, our spirits aligned.

We learn to embrace every scar, every tear,

For they tell our story, they make our purpose clear.

Shame has no power when love takes its place,

In the heart's vast expanse, it finds no space.

So, in the embrace of the dawning light,

Release the chains of Shame, and take your rightful flight.

For in this Courageous New Dawn we see,

The beauty of being, of living shame-free.

— P. LAST

44
UNYIELDING PRIDE: DAWN'S RESONANCE

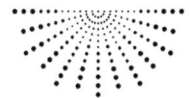

In the heart of the silent night,

Where dreams and doubts did once collide,

Emerges a strength, fierce and wide,

The feeling deep within – it's pride.

For every scar, every tear once cried,

In "Courageous New Dawn," they reside.

Not as reminders of times defied,

But badges of battles, undenied.

Past traumas faced, shadows cast aside,

Emotional triggers no longer our guide.

The inner child awakens, eyes open wide,

Finding joy in the journey, with pride as the ride.

To rise, to thrive, with stride and glide,

Not just to exist but to truly be alive.

In this dawn, our spirits confide,

The feeling resonating is unbreakable pride.

— P. LAST

45
EMERGENCE FROM SHADOWS: DAWN OVER DESPAIR

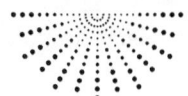

In the silent depths where despair does dwell,

Where hope's faint echoes seem distant as well,

A light emerges, piercing the gloom,

A courageous new dawn, making flowers bloom.

The night might be dark, the valley so deep,

Where whispers of sorrow make strong hearts weep,

Yet from the abyss, a strength does arise,

A will to push forward, to reach for the skies.

Despair, that old foe, with its weight so profound,

Can chain the spirit, making it bound.

But 'Courageous New Dawn' teaches us to see,

The power within to break free and just be.

Each tear that has fallen, each wound, and each scar,

It is a testament to battles, near and afar.

But as dawn breaks despair, with its radiant hue,

New horizons beckon, vistas anew.

For in the heart of darkness, when all seems forlorn,

A courageous spirit, anew, can be born.

With the might of the dawn, despair takes its leave,

As we learn once again, in ourselves to believe.

— P. LAST

LUMINANCE OF HOPE: THE DAWN'S ETERNAL SONG

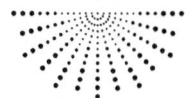

In the heart of the night, when all seems lost,

When dreams are distant and bridges are crossed,

There flickers a light, so subtle, so grand,

The feeling called 'Hope' that makes us withstand.

It whispers of futures, of what lies ahead,

It banishes nightmares and replaces dread.

With every sunrise that paints the sky,

Hope sings a song, teaching us to fly.

Amidst every storm, every trauma, every scar,

Hope is the compass, the guiding star.

For in "Courageous New Dawn," it plays a role,

Illuminating pathways, uplifting the soul.

Past pains are but echoes, shadows that cast,

Yet hope looks forward, freeing us from the past.

Embracing the now, with dreams to be spun,

Hope is the promise of battles to be won.

So when darkness beckons and challenges sprawl,

Let hope be the answer, the antidote to all.

For with every dawn, courageous and bright,

Hope ensures we're bathed in the most radiant light.

— P. LAST

47
DAWN'S REMEDY: BEYOND THE SHADOWS OF DOUBT

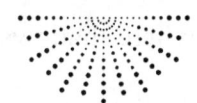

In the tender hues of the breaking morn,

Where light and shadow play and adorn,

Courageous New Dawn whispers a tale,

Of suspicion's grip, cold and frail.

With every rustle, every silent sigh,

Suspicion questions the who, what, and why.

Its heavy gaze, clouded and askew,

Seeks hidden motives in all that is true.

Yet, in the heart of this dawning day,

Lies a challenge, a brighter way,

To see beyond doubts that often bind,

And seek the truth with an open mind.

For Courageous New Dawn beckons us near,

To confront our suspicions, face our fear,

To trust once more in the world's grand design,

And let the heart's true light shine.

In the dance of doubt, where shadows play,

May we find clarity in the light of day.

For in every suspicion, every moment unsure,

Courageous New Dawn offers a cure.

— P. LAST

48
DAWN'S TRUST: THE BEACON OF HOPE

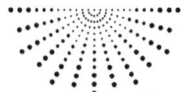

In the embrace of dawn, where whispers reside,

There lies a trust, vast as the tide.

For every shadow that dares to appear,

Courageous New Dawn casts away fear.

The weight of the past, its memories deep,

Are cradled in trust as the world stills to sleep.

And as day breaks, in its radiant light,

Trust in the promise that everything's right.

The bonds that we form, the dreams that we chase,

Are strengthened in trust, in its gentle embrace.

For in every heart, in every drawn breath,

Trust is the bridge between life and death.

With every challenge, every tear that's been shed,

Trust in the journey, the path that's ahead.

Courageous New Dawn, with its resolute might,

Kindles, the flame makes the future so bright.

So when the world's heavy and darkness is vast,

Look to the dawn; let go of the past.

For trust is the key, the hope that's reborn,

In every new day, in the Courageous New Dawn.

— P. LAST

49
AWAITING THE DAWN: THE PULSE OF ANTICIPATION

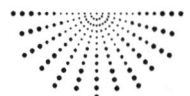

In the silent hush before the light,

There's a stirring, a pull, an eager might,

Anticipation fills the air so thick,

As the heart beats faster, the clock's tick quick.

For in the horizon, there lies a view,

Of a Courageous New Dawn, bold and true.

Each moment that leads to this bright array,

Holds promise and wonder, in night and day.

The heart's racing pulse, the eyes open wide,

At the cusp of the dream, where hopes reside.

Every past trauma, every deep scar,

Fuels the journey, propelling us far.

The inner child awakens, curious and free,

Gazing at what's to come, what's yet to be.

Mastering triggers, embracing the new,

Anticipation's song is a radiant hue.

As dawn approaches, the world starts to shift,

Giving power to dreams, a grandeur uplift.

Courageous New Dawn, with promise so grand,

Heralds a future where we, hand in hand,

Face all our tomorrows with strength and elation,

Rising, always rising, in sweet anticipation.

— P. LAST

50
DISGUST'S DANCE: DECIPHERING THE HIDDEN SONG

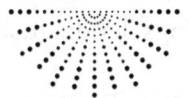

In the garden of feelings, where emotions enthrall,

Among joy and sorrow stands one quite tall.

Disgust, with its colors vivid and vile,

Challenges the heart to take an extra mile.

In the landscape of dawn, where courage does reign,

Such feelings, like disgust, leave an indelible stain.

Yet even in its grip, with disdain so profound,

A path to understanding is waiting to be found.

For in the heart of disgust, if we dare to peer,

Lies a protection mechanism, an ancient frontier.

Guarding us from harm, keeping threats at bay,

Yet often blinding us, leading us astray.

But with the Courageous New Dawn on the rise,

We see through the mirage, clear the cloudy skies.

Embrace this emotion without letting it steer,

For beneath its surface, deeper truths appear.

So in the dance of feelings, let disgust have its song,

But in the Courageous New Dawn, we learn to move along.

Recognizing its purpose, yet not letting it bind,

In this new era of growth, it's understanding we find.

— P. LAST

51
WHISPERS OF WONDER: THE DANCE OF DAWN AND SURPRISE

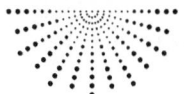

In the heart of the night, when all seemed askew,

There arose a moment, both wondrous and new.

It whispered of change, of tales yet untold,

Of Courageous New Dawns and futures so bold.

The stars blinked in wonder; the moon held its breath,

As surprise danced forth, dispelling the heath.

With twinkling eyes and a shimmering hue,

It sang of beginnings, of vistas anew.

Not a jolt in the dark or a gasp in the air,

But a gentle unfolding, light and rare.

The secrets it held, both ancient and vast,

Echoed tales of futures and shadows long past.

For the best of surprises, don't scream or shout,

They tiptoe in softly, casting out doubt.

And in Courageous New Dawn, where dreams intertwine,

Surprise is the sparkle, making souls shine.

Embrace the unexpected, let wonder seep in,

For in every fresh start, a journey begins.

In a world full of constants, routine, and known,

The gift of surprise makes our true growth shown.

— P. LAST

52
DAWN'S EMBRACE: A SYMPHONY OF GRATITUDE

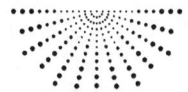

In the golden embrace of a courageous new day,

Gratitude whispers softly, showing the way,

To a heart open wide, to a soul so free,

In the dance of thanksgiving, we truly see.

For the lessons of past and traumas, we mend,

For emotional triggers that come to an end,

We're thankful, not just for the joy that's in sight,

But for darkness transformed, brought into the light.

The child within us, with wonder anew,

Sees the world with eyes that gratitude drew,

For every small miracle, for love's gentle song,

For the strength that emerges from battles long.

With every dawn that paints the sky,

Gratitude grows wings and teaches us to fly,

Over hurdles, through pain, beyond despair's night,

Into realms of hope, in pure, radiant light.

For the moments that heal, for the love that we share,

For the hands that support, for every prayer,

We rise, we thrive, with gratitude's embrace,

In the heart of dawn, finding our sacred space.

— P. LAST

53
EMERALD INSIGHTS: LESSONS FROM JEALOUSY'S HOLD

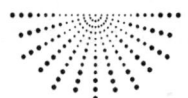

In the heart's vast chambers, where emotions reside,

Jealousy slinks in, with nowhere to hide.

Its venomous whispers, its envious glare,

A challenge for souls in need of repair.

Yet, within every shadow, a lesson awaits,

For the Courageous New Dawn never discriminates.

It beckons and calls, with a luminous hand,

Guiding us towards understanding so grand.

Jealousy, though potent, is a teacher, you see,

A mirror reflecting what we yearn to be.

But rather than drowning in its virulent tide,

We must seek the root, the reason it lied.

For in this brave dawn, we're equipped to explore,

The depths of our envy, its myths, and its lore.

To face every trigger, to mend every scar,

Reclaiming our power, no matter how far.

Awaken, dear soul, to the promise anew,

That with every green monster, there's a truth to construe.

By understanding its source, its enigmatic pull,

We dispel the illusions, making our hearts full.

So, in the Courageous New Dawn, let jealousy be,

A catalyst for growth, setting our spirits free.

For in this brilliant light, we discern and perceive,

The vastness of love we're destined to achieve.

— P. LAST

54
BOUNDLESS DAWN: THE ETERNAL EMBRACE OF LOVE

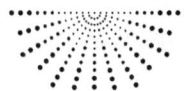

In the heart's vast expanse, a tale unfolds,

Of brave, boundless love, in whispers retold.

For in every pulse, every beat, and sigh,

There lies a dawn, a love that won't die.

A courageous new day, where love leads the way,

Shining brighter than stars, keeping darkness at bay.

With the strength of a thousand suns combined,

It's the beacon that guides when the world's unkind.

Past traumas may cloud, shadows may rise,

But love, undeterred, wears no disguise.

It conquers the tempest, the storm, and the night,

For in love's brave embrace, we find our true light.

Emotions may trigger, memories may sting,

Yet love's gentle touch makes the heart sing.

Reviving the innocence, the joy once known,

With love as our compass, we're never alone.

Awaken the child, that spirit so free,

Who knew love's pure magic, boundless and glee.

For in every challenge, love's call remains clear,

To rise, to thrive, and to hold what's dear.

So here's to the love, the journey, the dawn,

The courage to love, to keep moving on.

For in this grand tapestry, one truth stands above,

The mightiest force is the power of love.

— P. LAST

55
DANCE OF DAWN: EMBRACING FEAR'S GUIDING LIGHT

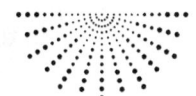

In the quiet corners where our fears reside,

There's a place where shadows and light coincide,

For even in the heart of the bravest, bold,

Lies a story of fear, untold.

But in the embrace of the Courageous New Dawn,

The shivers of dread begin to be drawn,

Out from their hiding into the day,

Where sunlight and courage wash them away.

Fear, a specter, an ancient old foe,

Whispers tales of woe, pulling us low.

Yet, in the brilliance of a new day's birth,

We find strength and the worth of our earth.

For Courageous New Dawn isn't just light,

It's the dance of the dark and bright, quite right.

It reminds us that fear, though real, is but a phase,

A moment, a challenge, a maze.

But with courage in heart and fire in the soul,

We face down our fears; we reach for the goal.

In the glow of the dawn, fear finds its place,

Not as a master but as a pace we embrace.

So let your fear come, let it teach, let it guide,

For in Courageous New Dawn, it won't hide.

Together, we face it, learn, and then strive,

In the face of our fears, we truly come alive.

— P. LAST

It's my sincere hope that the insights within these pages propel you toward continuous growth. Remember, nurturing a positive mindset isn't just beneficial—it's pivotal in sculpting a promising tomorrow. As you adapt to our new normal, do so with a renewed mindset.

Lastly, your feedback is invaluable. Sharing your reflections, critiques, or thoughts could inspire and guide another soul.

Your perspective is not just welcomed—it's essential. Your story might be the beacon someone needs to chase away their darkness.

Thank you.

Courageous New Dawn

If you got inspired while reading and would like to join a group of like-minded individuals on Facebook
HEALTHY BODY - HEALTHY MIND
at CommonSenseFactor.us

56
REFERENCE

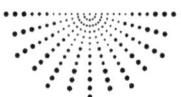

*H*ere is a list of various emotional feelings we've used to capture the poems in this book, but it's essential to remember that the human emotional spectrum is vast and can't be entirely captured in a list:

1. Afraid
2. Ashamed
3. Confident
4. Exhausted
5. Proud
6. Sad
7. Distracted
8. Frustrated
9. Surprised
10. Shocked
11. Worried

12. Embarrassed
13. Guilty
14. Shy
15. Angry
16. Happy
17. Nervous
18. Lonely
19. Confused
20. Overwhelmed
21. Joy
22. Sadness
23. Anger
24. Fear
25. Love
26. Jealousy
27. Gratitude
28. Surprise
29. Disgust
30. Anticipation
31. Trust
32. Suspicion
33. Hope
34. Despair
35. Pride
36. Shame
37. Guilt
38. Envy
39. Contentment
40. Boredom

41. Loneliness
42. Relief
43. Elation
44. Frustration
45. Apathy
46. Empathy
47. Confusion
48. Excitement
49. Indifference
50. Curiosity
51. Overwhelm
52. Embarrassment
53. Annoyance
54. Resentment
55. Nostalgia
56. Melancholy
57. Humiliation
58. Inspiration
59. Anxiety
60. Serenity

Many of these feelings can have nuances or subcategories and can be experienced differently by individuals based on their life experiences, cultures, and personal perspectives.

www.ingramcontent.com/pod-product-compliance
Lightning Source LLC
Chambersburg PA
CBHW060032040426
42333CB00042B/2312